Foot Care

Caring for Your Feet – Heart and "Sole"

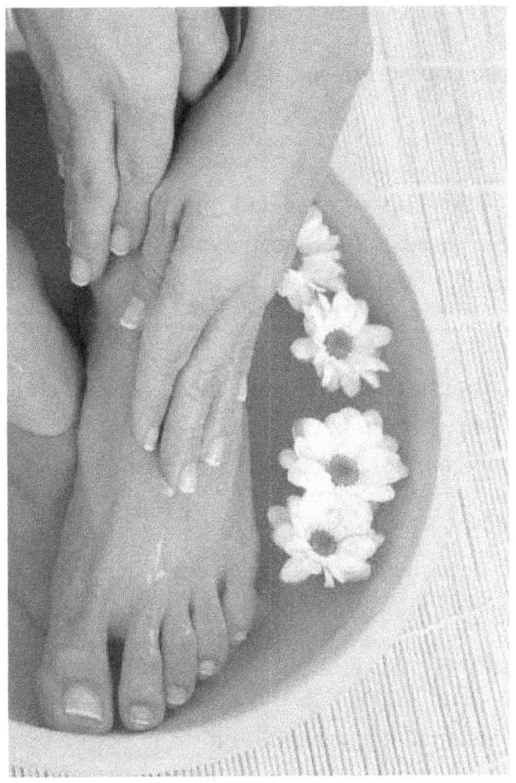

Healthy Learning Series

Dueep Jyot Singh

Mendon Cottage Books

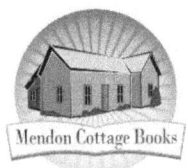

JD-Biz Publishing

All Rights Reserved.

Disclaimer

Warning

Our books are available at

1. Amazon.com
2. Barnes and Noble
3. Itunes
4. Kobo
5. Smashwords
6. Google Play Books

Table of Contents

Introduction 5

Design of Your Feet 7

Proper Footwear 10

Problems Due to High Heels 15

Noticed the high heels? 19

Health Concerns about Wearing High Heels 21

Back, Knee, Shoulder and Foot Pain 22

Heel Problems 25

Foot Problems 27

Bunions and Bursitis 27

Corns and Calluses 28

Athlete's Foot 30

Ingrown Toenails 32

Back Pain 33

Achilles Tendinitis 35

Claw Toes 36

Morton's Neuroma 36

Tips for Buying Proper Footwear 37

Natural Footcare 41

Oatmeal Scrub 41

Healing Cracked Heels..41

Softening Soles 43

Conclusion 45

Author Bio..47

Publisher..58

Introduction

Our feet to have supported and carried us all our lives walking an average of 70,000 miles in the process! This book is going to tell you all about how to take care of your feet, common problems, and feet care.

Did you know that your feet are the key to the rest of your body? Unfortunately, we have a tendency of neglecting our feet, although we may spend thousands in beautifying the rest of our body. However, the poor feet are just given a cursory pedicure and massage. And that is that, we are done with them.

The ancient Egyptians, Chinese and Indians observed that the tension in any part of the foot would be capable of mirroring tension in a corresponding part of the body.

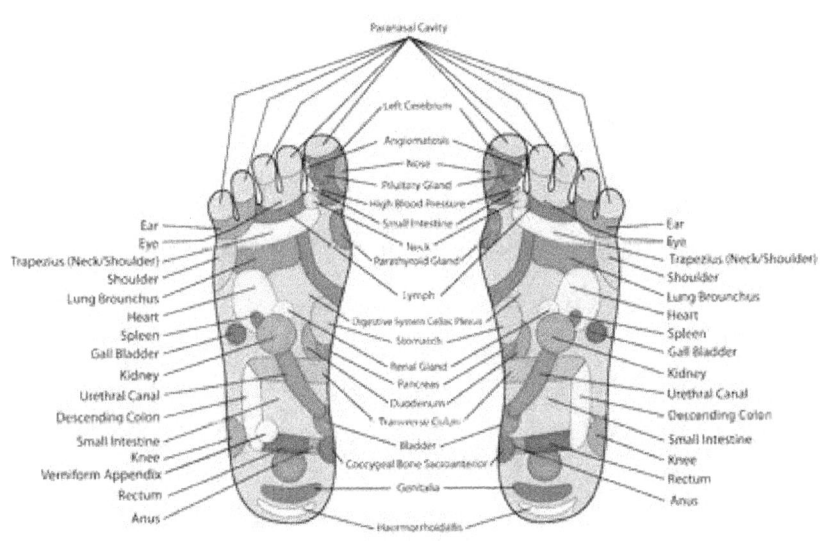

I remember as a child suffering badly from myopia. Our family ophthalmologist advised my father – press the pads of her feet, just beneath her toes. If they hurt or ache, there is a chance that her eyes can be brought back to 20/20 vision, because she is still a child. If they are solid, I am sorry, I cannot do anything about it then.

This was in the early seventies. I remember my father coming back enthusiastically and pressing the tender pads under my toes, – the ball of the foot – asking me if there was any sort of feeling or sensation there. Nah, I said, because I was not one to make a fuss, even though that pressure was aching slightly. But father took that as truth and that is why he took it for granted that his child would be wearing huge glasses throughout her life.

As far as I know, that ophthalmologist was using some acupuncture theory, and I am not sure, what he intended to do about my eyesight, if I had yelled, "my feet ache, especially when you press them." I do not know if there is any scientific basis about pressure points in the feet having corresponding pressure points in the rest of the body, but for centuries people have believed in this assertion.

Thus, according to this theory when you treat your big toes, there is going to be a related effect in the head and treating your whole foot is going to have a relaxing and relieving effect on your whole body.

This is the reason why traditional massage always talks about massaging your feet with warm oil so that the whole body can relax.

Keeping your feet healthy is no laughing matter. So here are some tips and techniques, which are going to help you keep these important organs fit, fine and in good working condition for the rest of your lives.

Design of Your Feet

Bones of the Human Foot

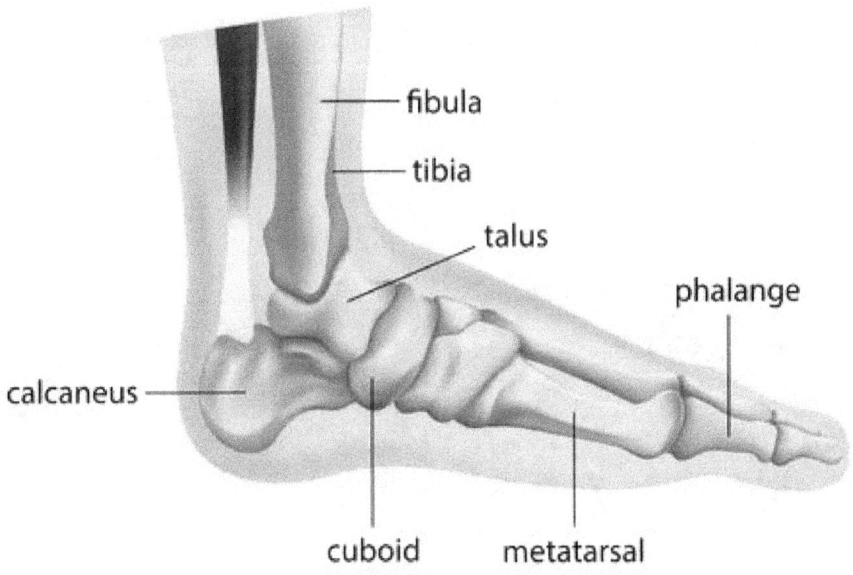

Your feet have been designed by nature to act as a pliable platform. This is going to support your body weight in an upright posture. It is also going to act as a lever to propel the body forward while walking, jumping and running.

The human foot has thus been designed in the form of elastic arches. You can also call this design to be a shock absorber, in the form of springs.

In ancient times we stimulated reflexes naturally by walking bare feet over stones, rough grounds and rocks. But nowadays, we have lost much of nature's way of maintaining a balanced and healthy natural reflexology on our pressure points because our feet are covered with soft footwear.

When we were children, we were brought up to wake up early in the morning and walk barefoot in the dewy grass till the sun rose. According to my grandmother, this was the practice of ancients to keep the younger generation healthy. I have a feeling, that that barefoot dancing in the grass in the early morning was nothing more than our pressure points getting massaged by the cushiony grass. Also, we were touching mother Earth with our bare feet.

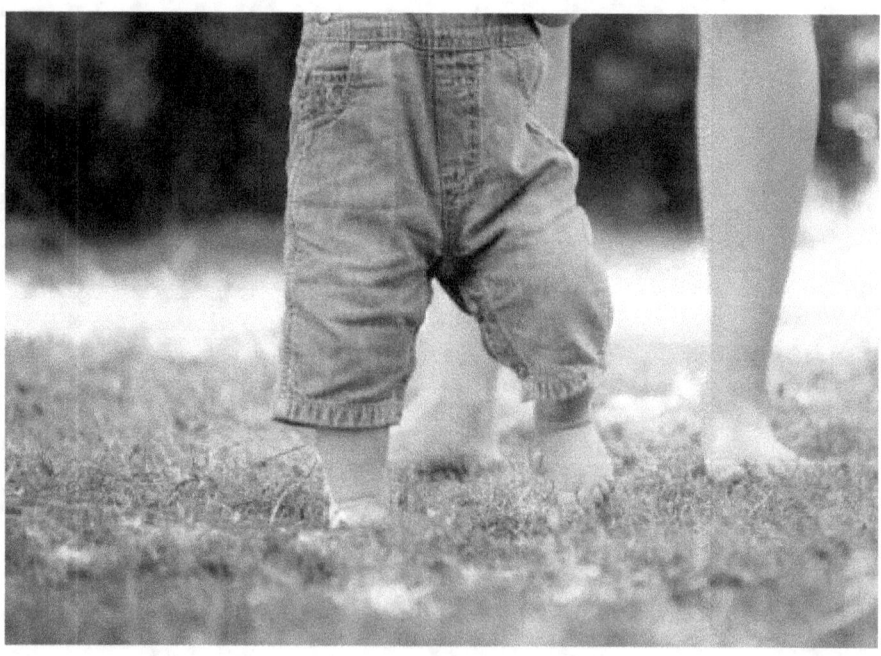

Incidentally, this practice kept us healthy throughout our childhood. Unfortunately, as we grew up, we became more indolent, and we were not going to leave our comfortable beds at the break of dawn just to walk in the grass. We would rather have our alarm clock wake us up, because we have this hard day at the office ahead.

And that is why, we grew susceptible to a number of stress-related diseases, because the stress and tension in our bodies had not been sloughed away during our morning walk.

This is a fact, and even if scientists are still researching on whether it is true or not, you can take it as truth. So try walking barefoot on the grass, in the early morning for about an hour or so, and see the amazing change in your state of health.

Proper Footwear

A number of top shoe manufacturers are using the science of reflexology for designing shoe products. I went to an exhibition where a vendor on acupuncture was selling shoes and slippers with pressure points built in them.

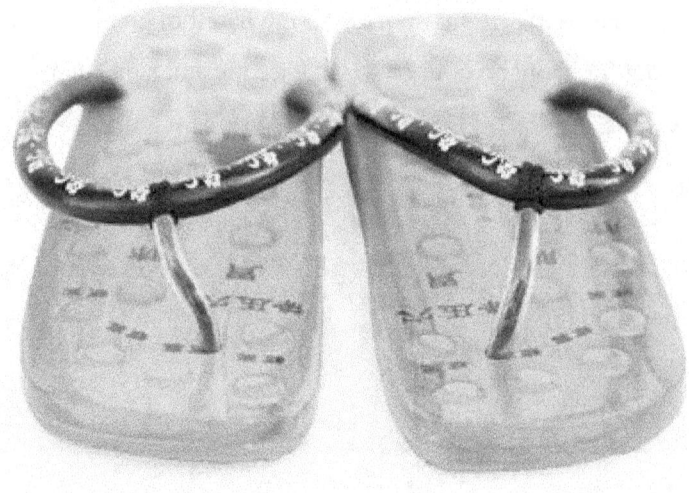

All you have to do was walk in these slippers throughout the day and the gentle points would press in the corresponding points of your feet, as soon as pressure was put on them, the moment you put your feet down to walk.

Those shoes/slippers sold like hot cakes. I could not manage to grab a pair, but even if it is a fad or not, this is one product which is very popular in our part of the world. These slippers are normally made in China and sold here! I do not know whether they have managed to make their presence felt anywhere else in the world, but I think it is a pretty good idea.

Nowadays, shoes can be considered to be a symbol of self-esteem and status along with jeans, jewelry, designer clothes, and other symbols of the modern and fashionable stylish lifestyle.

When designer clothes, jeans and jewelry have become uniformly blah and repetitive, it is possible that your footwear may set you apart from the maddening crowd. I am not very fashion conscious, but when I was at college, I had my own particular uniform. It was made up of a snow white shirt, a blue silk scarf, blue jeans and flying boots up to my knee.

It made me look like a Cossack warrior,[1] and surprisingly enough, 60% of the students were so impressed by that outfit, that they began hunting the city for flying boots! Within three months, the college rang with the sound of clomping flying boots.

Even men down the ages have been fascinated by different types of footwear, which reflect style, taste, and also the attention paid to small details and also one's sense of self-esteem.

---

[1] Incidentally, this outfit earned me the nickname of "Khan Saheb" given to me by my teachers! That meant Khan Sir, because according to them, I looked like a rough and tough warrior like Pakhtoon from Afghanistan, of proud mien and conquering master of all I surveyed! This was before the Russian invasion of Afghanistan.

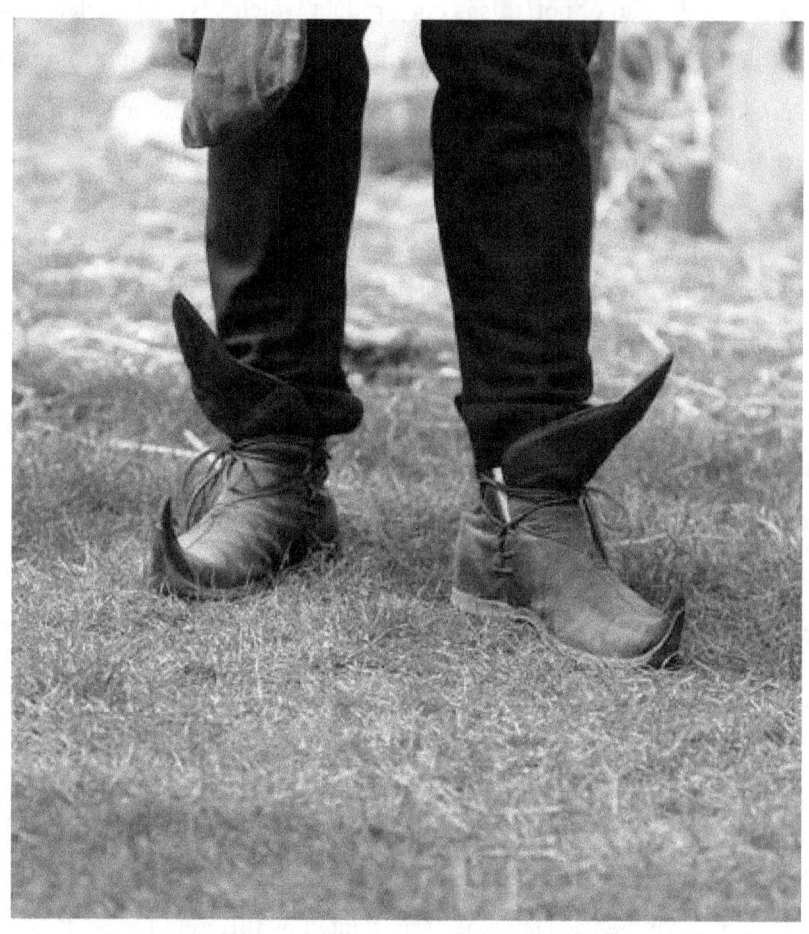

In medieval times, shoes were curled at the tips, and the more intricate the curls were, the more important that person was in society. In fact, sometimes the curls were so large, that a person could not move comfortably. Talk about affectations! The Romans wore their sturdy Roman sandals made out of leather, which were so comfortable that they could walk miles in them. And traditional deerskin moccasins have come down from the ages to protect the feet of the Native Americans.

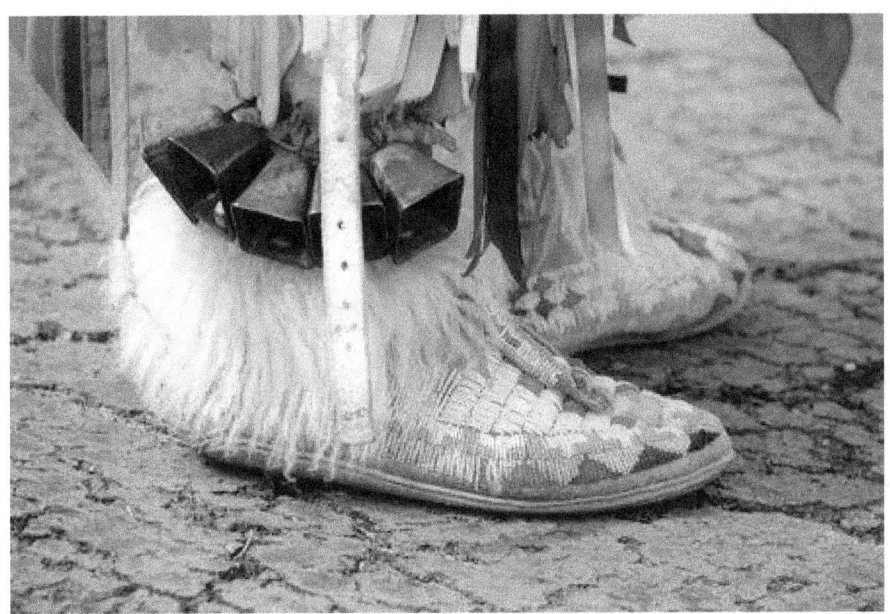

Like I said at one time the use of stylish and costly footwear was associated with status, especially when Queen Elizabeth the first had tiny shoes with diamond studded heels! Small feet were supposed to be the sign of dainty aristocracy, and she was very proud of her little feet.

One of her preserved shoes is supposed to be as small as a child's shoe. Golly! I would rather call that particular small size misshapen for a lady about 5'4" which incidentally was considered to be tall in her times. She was described to be tall, with slender fingers, and with a tiny waist and tiny feet.

Just imagine a grown-up hale and hearty woman walking about on such tiny feet further restricted in such small shoes. No wonder the courtiers of that time winced whenever they walked because their shoes must have pinched them terribly!

However, we in the 21st century can be considered lucky, because we have such a wide-ranging choice of excellent and high-quality footwear which cares more about protecting our feet than about being a fashionable two sizes too small!

Problems Due to High Heels

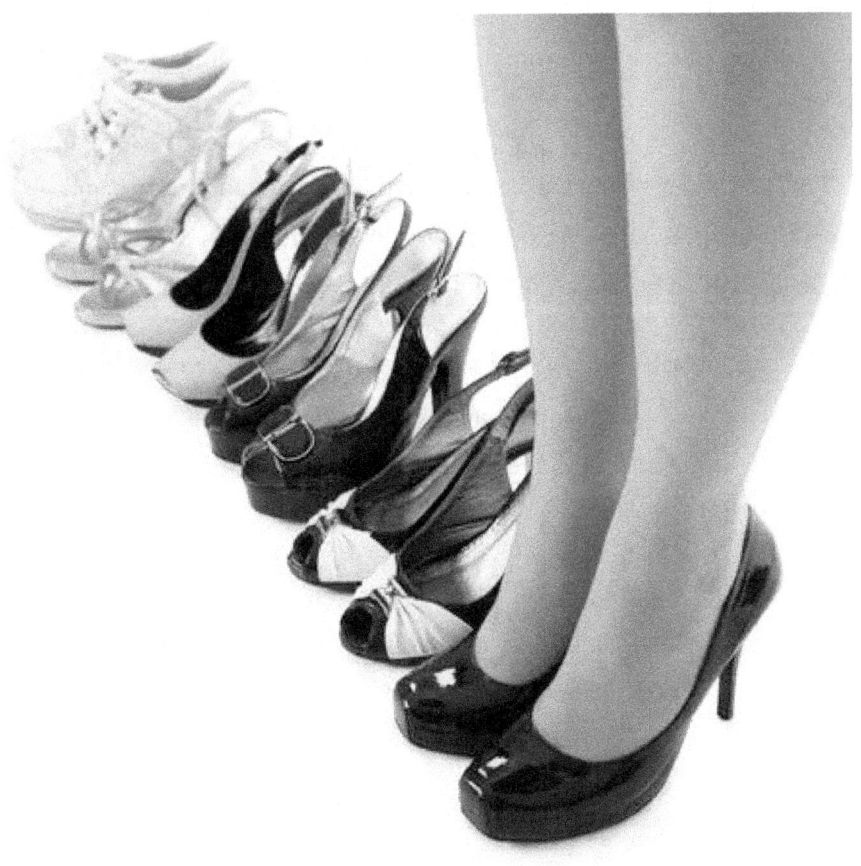

I remember one of my favorite writers writing about high heels in one of her books. The heroine has just come back from a party, where she had worn high-heeled shoes. She describes them as being designed by a designer who hated women. He had found the best way to torture them, by creating footwear which seriously hurt their feet so much.

Nevertheless, it is a matter of vanity, which makes women wear high heels. Nobody really expects men to make a drastic fashion statement in footwear. You may not find 21st-century men wearing high heels, even though it was a fashionable fashion statement in the sixteenth and seventeenth centuries. But then at that time the men wore them only to levees or balls when they did not have to walk much.

But a 21st-century woman is also going to be looking for creative and interesting fashion designs in footwear. And naturally, as they are so much in demand, high heels are going to be an important part of these designs.

Why are high heels the type of footwear which are most controversial and always under scrutiny, dispute and discussion? That is because vanity in women does not allow the admission of wearing something which is so painful to the feet.

Catherine de Medici can be blamed for these instruments of torture, because she was very short. Her shoes were wooden with the heels raised about 5 cm above the 25 mm platform sole.

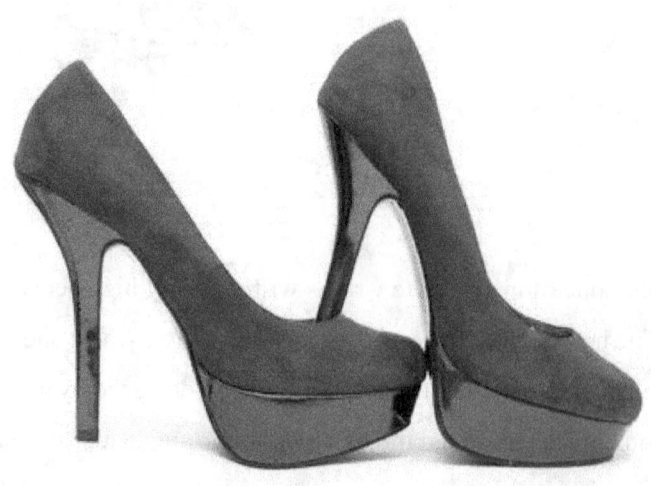

But as time went by, the heels began to be raised to heights of about 10 cm. They may also have narrow tips, which one calls pencil heels. And just like fragile pencils, they snap off at the slightest provocation.

One of the rare times I wore high heels was a time when I had to walk on the catwalk at a fashion show because according to my fashion designer colleague and best friend – who was managing the show, – high heels helped all of us models to walk like professional models from the hip.

They do. They also garner you Wolf whistles from the audience and sighs of envy because they create the illusion of long, long legs. Also, your ankles look so slender in those silk stockings and your feet look tiny. However, the whole problem is that you have to be very careful about your center of gravity and sense of balance.

I managed to cross the catwalk, and at the end of the program, when I was walking towards the changing rooms one of those heels got stuck in one of the cracks between the floorboards. And it snapped off, while I took a graceful tumble earthwards. [2]

I did not measure myself full length on my face on the floor, but when I got up from my knees, the first thing I did was take off those shoes and throw them at the nearest wall with lots of bad language. As far as I know, they

---

[2] At such special moments and occasions, don't expect any of your friends to rush up to you to help you up. They are too busy hooting with laughter at your discomfiture. Some of them may even ask an encore thinking that you did it on purpose. The only ones who are going to be sympathetic with you are the ones who can say proudly – Been There Done That!

may still be there with my worst wishes. It took around three weeks for that twisted ankle to heal.

And I promised myself never ever to wear those silly things again, however, much my best friends persuaded me that I needed to wear them while swaying on the catwalk.

And then about 11 years later, just a week ago, I had to go to a party. So I decided to dust off my old stylish high heels, and get my feet into them. I definitely did not enjoy the party in the initial stages of the party.

That was because five minutes of walking and my feet had begun to complain and whimper. My toes would soon have blisters. My sense of balance in high heels had been lost in the 11 years, which had passed since my last essay into the world of high heels.

So I enjoyed my party, sitting out in the most comfortable sofa without circulating among the standing partygoers. All the men were sensibly clad in flat shoes. All the women were in stylish high heels. And when I limped home, and took off those terrible tortuous fashion statements, the first thing I did was put my poor, swollen feet into a basin full of hot water, one spoonful of salt and 1 tablespoon full of mustard oil.

I soaked them for 20 minutes to get rid of the pain, aches and ensuing swelling. After that I picked up my feet out of that soothing and now lukewarm solution and extended them to an angle of 90° from my sitting position. I kept them in this position – neither higher, neither lower, – for another 20 minutes and so I got my feet back into their normal un-swollen pain-free condition.

This incidentally was a remedy given to me by one of my professional model friends who, poor thing, had to do every day, because she had to wear high heels day in day out. Talk about torture, and then the most effective antidote for this torture. How we like to suffer in the name of vanity...

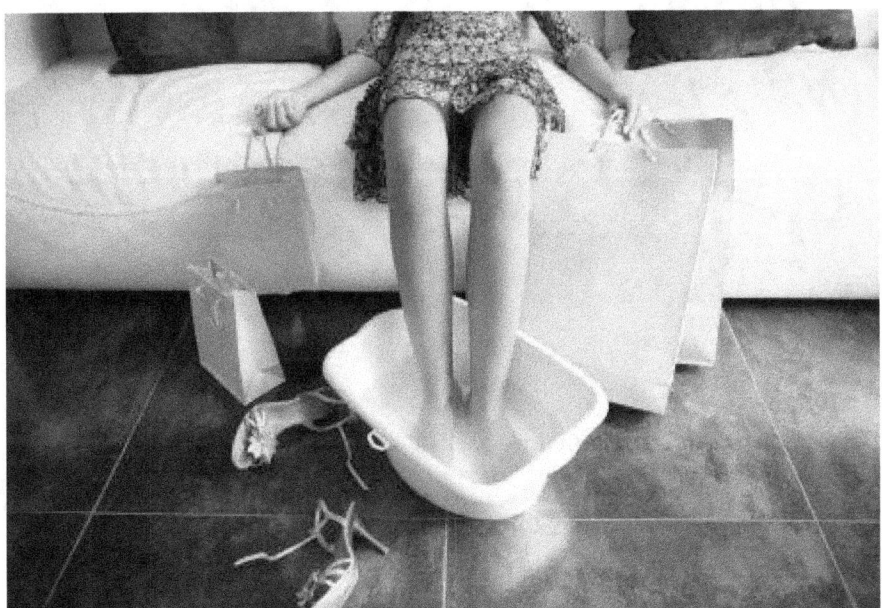

Noticed the high heels?

Gone are the days when heels were just black or brown in color. Nowadays fashion designers have become so particular about alluring and irresistible designer heels that you can get all sorts of matching heels with the designs being created by the designers.

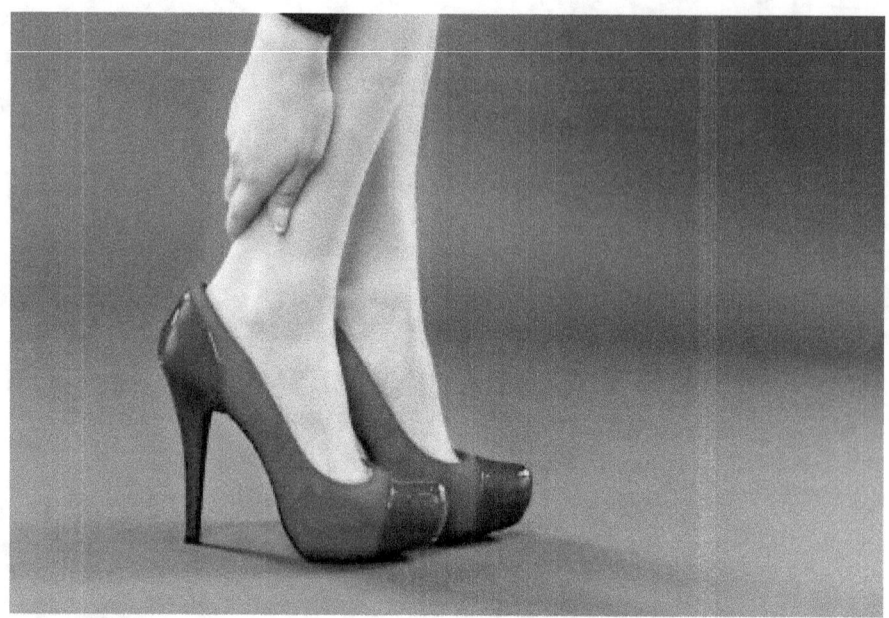

However here are the health drawbacks which heels are going to cause.

High-heeled footwear is going to throw the entire weight of the user forward. That makes it more difficult for him to sustain an upright balance. Furthermore these shoes are going to put abnormal pressure and excessive force on the ball of the foot compared to the shoes that men wear. In such well-made shoes worn by men, the foot is almost parallel to the ground.

But in the high-heeled shoes preferred by women, the arches are raised abnormally high, the heels raise the heels of the feet and thus the whole pressure is placed on the frontal portion of the foot. So they are bad when you are standing, but they are definitely going to be worse while you are walking.

Instead of placing your full foot on the ground, you are placing the ball of the foot first and the rest of the foot is still in the air because it has been supported by the shoe's heel. Once upon a time, the whole weight of the body was taken up by the whole foot placed steadily on the ground. But now, you are placing the weight on about one third of the whole foot, the frontal portion. No wonder it begins to squeak in despair, after just a couple of minutes of walking.

These heels are also going to force you to use a lot of extra and unnecessary muscular effort to keep yourself from falling flat on your face. The bones of our feet are designed by nature to be on a certain plane and the moment you wear high heels, this certain plane and design is disrupted.

Health Concerns about Wearing High Heels

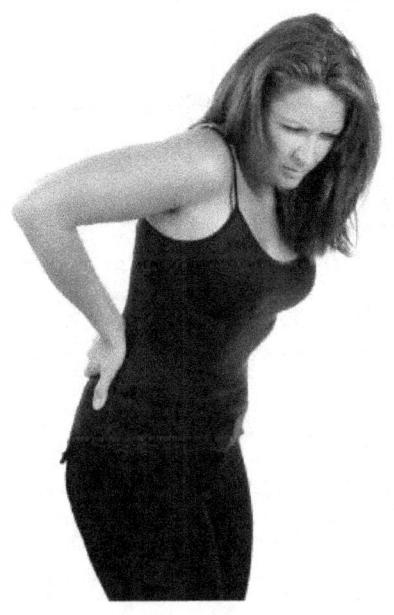

Gynecologists, orthopedists chiropractors as well as fitness instructors especially in the USA are all unanimous on one point that is that high heels are bad for health. Even though high heels signify style, or fashionable haute couture, walking on these high heels are going to put 25% greater force on the knee than walking barefoot.

These statistics have been taken from the American orthopedic foot and ankle society and the Harvard Medical School, which suggests that women should wear shoes with the heels of no more than 6 cm and even these should be worn for not more than two – 3 hours a day. That is in case you find it really necessary to wear heels. They would rather that you wear flat – soled shoes.

It is true that standing in high heels make you look taller, with your behind sticking out and the natural curvature of the spine looks so attractive and great. But these high heels are going to alter the curvature of the spine in the opposite direction. It is also going to create a hunch in the lower back.

That is why, based on these serious researched reports, you should indulge in high-heeled shoes only on special occasions when you don't have to walk around too much or stand for long. Besides this, never wear them if you are expecting. Apart from the wobbly center of gravity and unsteadiness of high heels, there is always the chance that you might trip on those unreliable pencil heels.

Back, Knee, Shoulder and Foot Pain

A number of women have been blaming their high heels for back shoulder and foot pain. In many cases, they are ignoring other serious medical conditions. This pain can be viewed to overweight or due to bad posture. It can also be due to other related or unrelated medical problems.

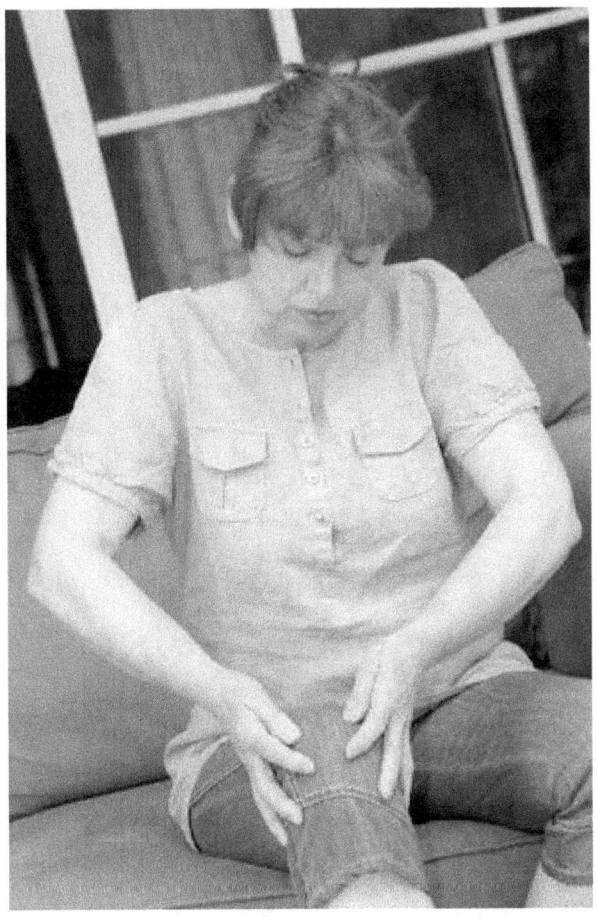

For instance knee pains invariably arise from the joint between the kneecap and the lower end of the thigh bone. This is called the femur. This patello–femoral joint has a number of peculiar characteristics, which are gender related. That is why women athletes who subject their knees to high stress are always going to develop anterior knee pain.

Also, women have been naturally fashioned to bear children and that is why nature has made the pelvic region broader for women. Apart from this, they are also going to have ligaments getting lax with the passage of time and the influence of female hormones. These are the anatomical and physiological factors which are going to dispose women to suffer from knee pain.

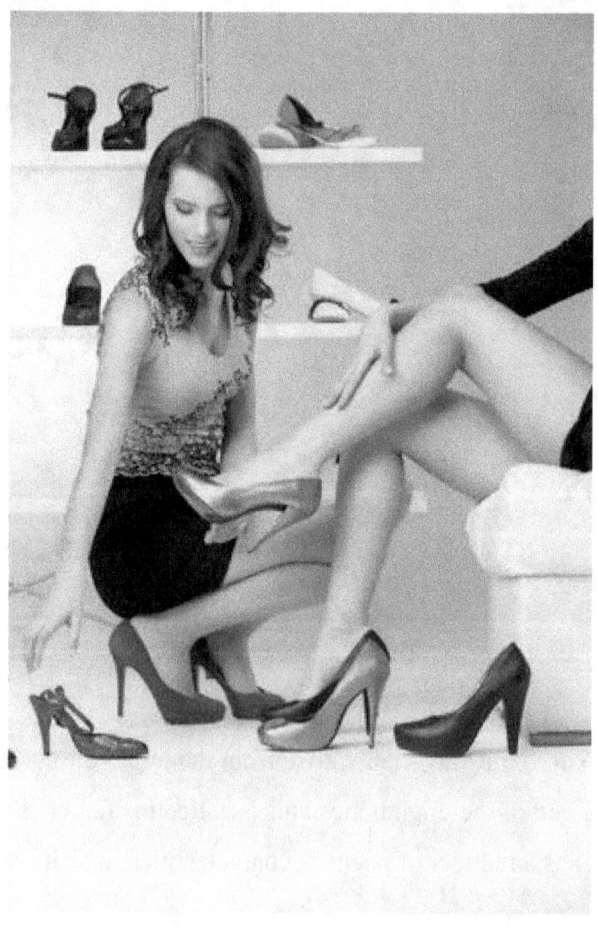

But you blame that pain on your high heels. Also, women following a sedentary lifestyle without plenty of exercise are going to gain weight. *All these are going to impose loads up to seven times of your body weight on your kneecaps.* So imagine you with that overweight load on your feet, which have been jammed into high heels.

Your poor kneecap which is endowed with the thickest articular cartilage in the body is going to give way under this extra weight with absolutely no support from the foot. So if you have knee problems, you may want to get rid of the heels as well as shed extra weight. This is going to relieve the load on your kneecap joint exponentially.

Heel Problems

All feet are not alike. Feet can either be supple or rigid flat or normally arched. Different kind of feet are going to need different types of shoes

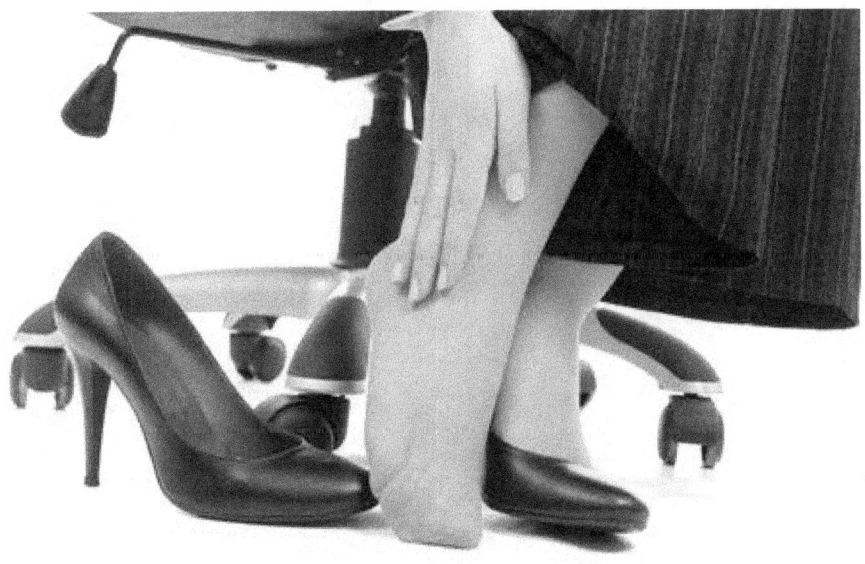

Shoes provide your feet with protection and support but the wrong type of shoes can put pressure on the wrong places. They are thus going to cause itching pain and deformities and can also put the stymie on your stepping outside style.

Ill fitting shoes covered with moisture are going to cause friction, which are going to further on cause sores. That is why people who indulge in lots of marching make sure that their socks are powdered well so that there is absolutely no sweat, on their feet, which can cause sores on their feet.

At least these modern soldiers are not like the Zulus, who ran 30 miles and at the end of the run were ready for war. They ran barefoot!

With the heights of shoes soaring, doctors are reporting an increase in foot injuries, broken ankles, sprained feet, and fractures of bones. As my half farcical example given above, just the snapping off of my shoe heel causing me to sprain my ankle but it could easily have been a bone fracture.

Uncomfortable and impractical footwear are going to give rise to a number of foot ailments, which include calluses, corns, fatigue, bunions, backache, athlete's foot, ingrown toenails, bursitis, claw toes, arthritis knees, sprained ankles, and Achilles Tendinitis .

Oh my, you say, all these foot problems? Yes and all of them could be avoided only if you stop wearing those pesky heels.

Foot Problems

Bunions and Bursitis

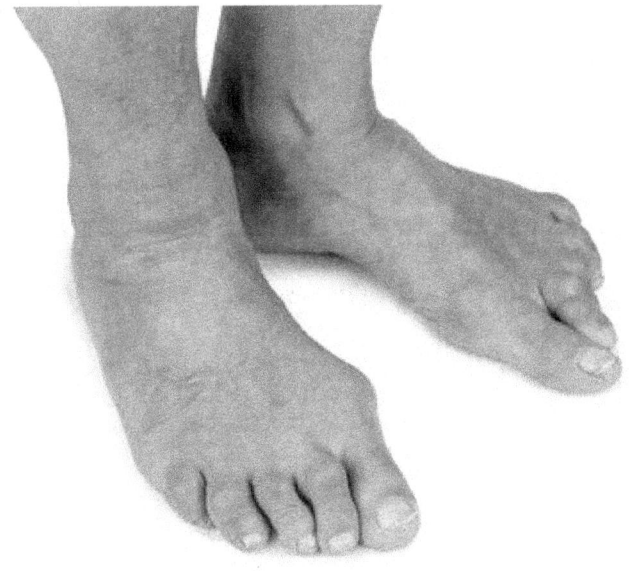

Bunions are normally characterized by prominent bumps on the inside of your foot these are normally found around the big toe and are more common in women.

People with an inherited weakness in the toe joints are going to get them and ill fitting shoes are going to worsen this problem

One result of bunions is that the bony base of your twisted big toe is going to be pushed out beyond the normal outline of your foot. It is going to form an unsightly bump known as a bunion.

Sometimes persistent pressure of tight shoes are going to cause pain under the pressure point. This is known as bursitis.

In addition, the affected joint can develop osteoarthritis sooner than it normally would. If you have developed bursitis to in your foot, you can relieve the pressure on the bunion by cutting a hole in the top of an old shoe. Wear it until the inflammation clears up.

I remember my grandmother doing that. She had bunions on both her big toes. She immediately cut out holes in her best leather shoes – much to my horror, and dismay – and that she was with those bunions poking out in an unsightly manner from the side of the shoes. But she was of a quality to carry off anything with a high hand!

If the bunion is severe, you may have to get a surgical operation done to straighten out your big toe.

Corns and Calluses

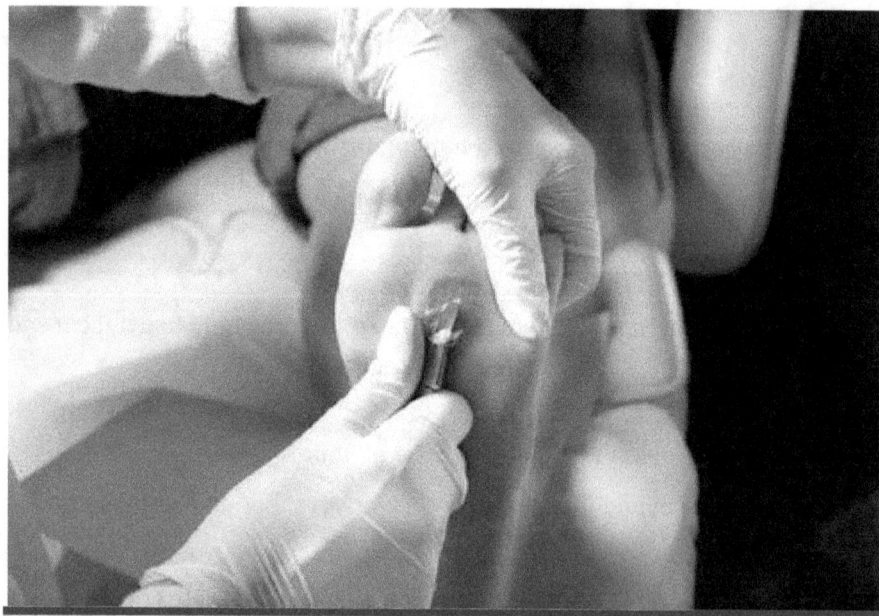

These are normally going to form when dead skin cells harden and thicken all over an area of the foot. This is a defense against excessive pressure and friction. They are usually found on the ball of the foot, the heels, the inside of the big toe, and the soles of the feet.

I remember my father going on a tour where the hosts had spread themselves out to impress my father and his inspection team.

He spent an once-in-a-lifetime week at that place, with gourmet food and liquor flowing – because the hosts wanted him to pass a multimillion dollar contract, which he did not because the quality of their product was substandard –. Anyway, when he came back and described the trip to his children, we asked him whether he had enjoyed the good food and the drink. He had not. He was suffering from a corn!

When we asked him that all he had to do was call out to any of the hotel employees for a corn plaster, he blinked a little at this easy solution. He had never suffered from corns before! And he did not know that it was so easy to get rid of them!

Naturally, we more worldly wise kids were extremely amused at the rather innocent and simple nature of our father, who kept wondering what caused his feet to pain so much. That was because he had always been well clad while walking in his 40 years of traipsing up and down mountains and had never suffered from foot problems! So one tiny corn and his trip was ruined!

However, as we youngsters had met them often during our Marching, parade and PT sessions during cadet training, we knew that the moment we got any sort of corn, we changed our shoes and put on a corn plaster. Also, we prevented the formation of blisters by putting on socks which were well powdered especially when we had to go on long training marches with heavy knapsacks on our backs.

So here are the tips for getting relief of corns.

Change the shoes and wear those which are going to fit you more comfortably.

Soften the skin with a scrubber during your bath. After that, put a small spongy rubber ring around the corn, if you don't have a corn plaster handy.

Remember that if you are suffering from diabetes mellitus **do not use** a razor to peel off the thickened skin. This is a normal method in which many people cut the thickened skin.

Athlete's Foot

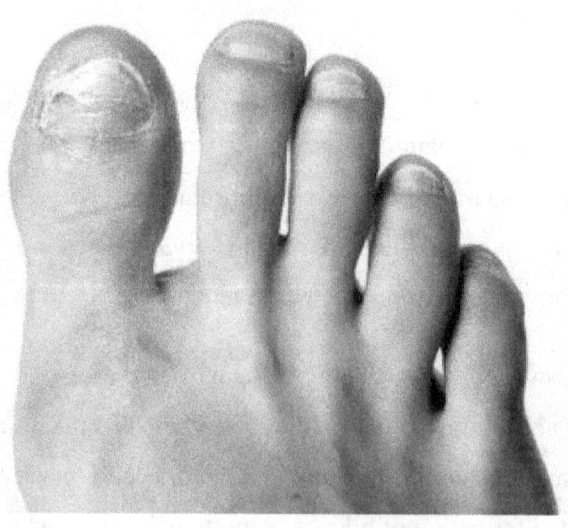

In this condition, a fungus is going to grow in the skin between and under the toes, especially the fourth and fifth toes. The skin is going to become red, itchy, and flaky.

A moist atmosphere, especially the presence of water or sweat is going to make the top layer of skin soggy and white. The fungus is also going to affect other parts of the nail and the foot. The nails are going to become yellow and thickened.

Athlete's foot is highly contagious, and is contracted in showers, dressing rooms, gyms, swimming pool, lockers, and other warm and damp areas where fungus can thrive. Men are more affected than women.

It is also going to flourish in moist atmospheres, especially when you have not change your shoes or socks for a while. This reminds me of one particular amusing incident in the interesting life and times of yours faithfully.

When in service, Father suffered from athlete's foot, which made all his toenails deformed and yellow. So did all his colleagues! That was because that area was particularly muggy and moist.

The doctors in that particular base knew all about this very prevalent affliction of which all their officers and men suffered. So they gave them an ointment which was sulfur based to get rid of the fungus. It worked.

They were also told not to wear shoes and socks for a couple of months and go to work in open mouthed sandals and slippers so that their toes could get a chance to breathe.

So it was very hilarious, seeing everybody in pristine, formal uniform worn with sandals. And as everyone from the top man to the most junior man was in sandals or in slippers, nobody hauled them up for not being in proper uniform! So here are the tips learned from father on how you can prevent athlete's foot.

1. Maintain good foot hygiene by washing and drying your feet completely, especially if they are wet or you have just taken a bath.

2. After you have taken off your shoes and socks, allow your feet to dry in the air to get rid of all the sweat.

3. Keep your feet dry by wearing absorbent socks made of natural fiber. These include cotton socks or bamboo fiber socks.

4. Wear shoes with porous soles and open sandals.

5. There are a number of antifungal creams, or powders which you need to apply if the skin is soggy. Dry the skin out with a liberal application of antifungal powder.

Ingrown Toenails

This is a common debilitating condition which is usually going to afflict your large toe. It is caused by poor foot hygiene ill fitting shoes and injury to your nails.

There are many options for the treatment of this condition. These are going to include getting your doctor to treat them. You will also need to take preventive measures and precautions so that they do not recur.

The only time I suffered from ingrown toenails was about two decades ago when I had to wear uniform shoes. These were not quite comfortable, and they were tight against the toe. Eight hours of waiting those shoes, and pressure being put on the large toe, I soon found that a portion of the nails had begun growing inwards.

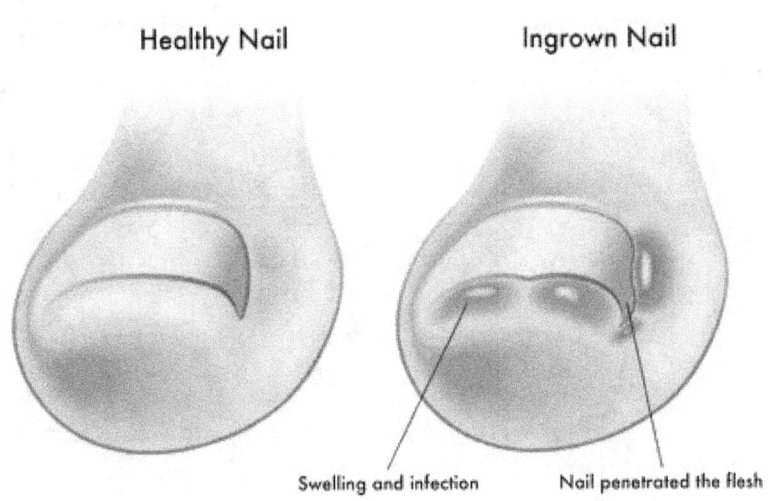

Healthy Nail	Ingrown Nail
	Swelling and infection Nail penetrated the flesh

That painful condition was relieved by my podiatrist who told me to get rid of those shoes, immediately. He also told me to trim my nails properly so that I never suffered from this problem again.

This is when I began to get more interested in foot conditions, especially those brought about through sheer inertia, laziness, and a flippant attitude.

Back Pain

It has been calculated that more than three quarters of the world's population are going to experience back pain at some time or the other in their lives. Did you know that in the West, low back pain is the most common cause of illnesses related absence from work?

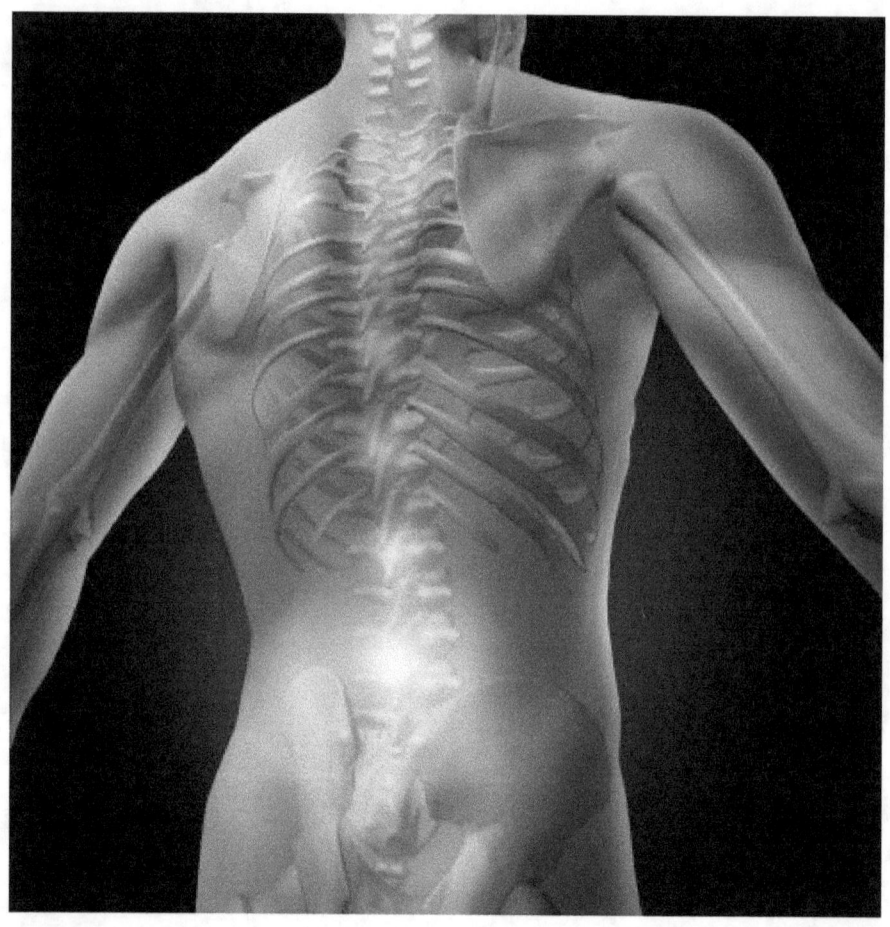

When your job requires you to stand on your feet for long periods, you are going to run the risk of getting backaches and varicose veins. So look at the shoes you are wearing. If they are high heels, they are the natural culprits. Do they really fit you? If you are standing for a number of hours on ill fitting shoes, with high heels, you have made yourself vulnerable to backache.

Achilles Tendinitis

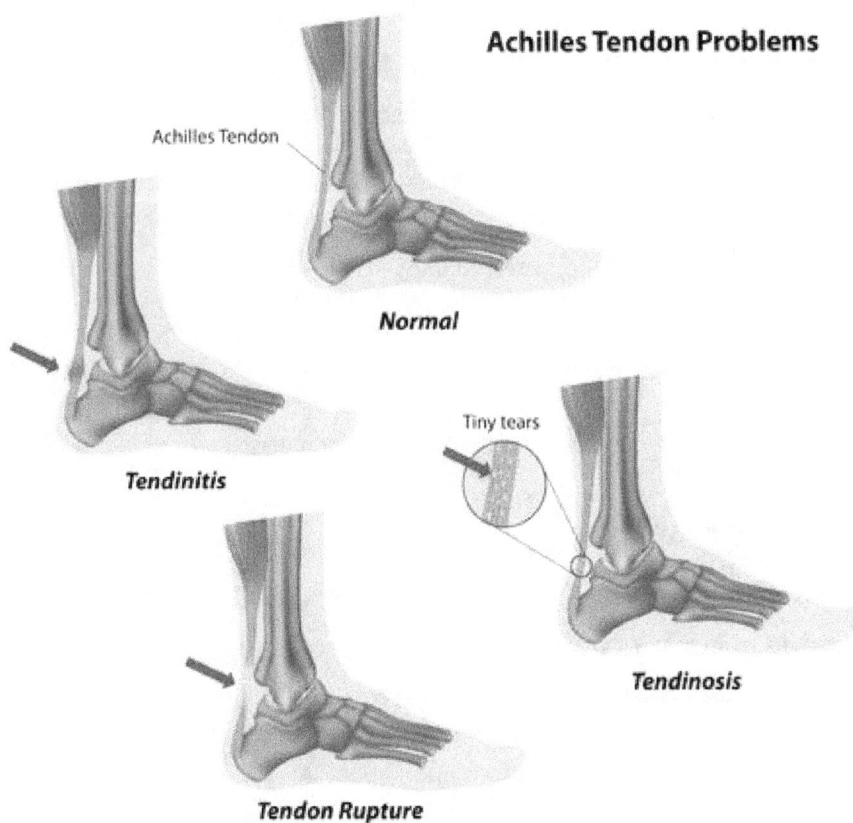

The Achilles tendon is present at the back of your ankle. But shoes are going to cause injuries to that particular region. The Achilles tendon attaches the muscles of the calf to the heel bone. It is one of the strongest of tendons in the body. Any injury to this tendon is going to result in your feet unable to move. You are also going to suffer from hind foot pain.

In ancient times, warriors used to hamstring their opponents and prisoners by cutting the Achilles tendons. Thus, they rendered them incapable of escaping because these people were now lame forever.

Claw Toes

A claw toe is contracted when severe pressure is applied on the middle and end joints in a toe. These normally result from a muscular imbalance that causes the ligaments and tendons to become unnaturally tight. So your toe is going to get crooked and resemble a claw. That is because the joint is curling downwards.

Arthritis can also be a reason for claw toes. So change the type of your footwear to get rid of the pain and discomfort of a claw toe.

Morton's Neuroma

This is a neural condition of the interdigital nerves. This condition normally occurs in women who wear ill fitting shoes, especially if they are middle-aged.

You can get more interesting information about this particular condition on this URL –

http://www.foothealthfacts.org/footankleinfo/mortons-neuroma.htm

Tips for Buying Proper Footwear

I have heard about people who go crazy when they are confronted with shoes, and buy about 6 to 12 pairs at one time in one huge shopping binge. I do not know the mental workings behind such an obsession. Though we could understand why Eva Peron and Imelda Marcos had more than hundred pairs of shoes. That was because they were forced to go barefoot in childhood, due to circumstances and that hunger rankled in their subconscious throughout their lives.

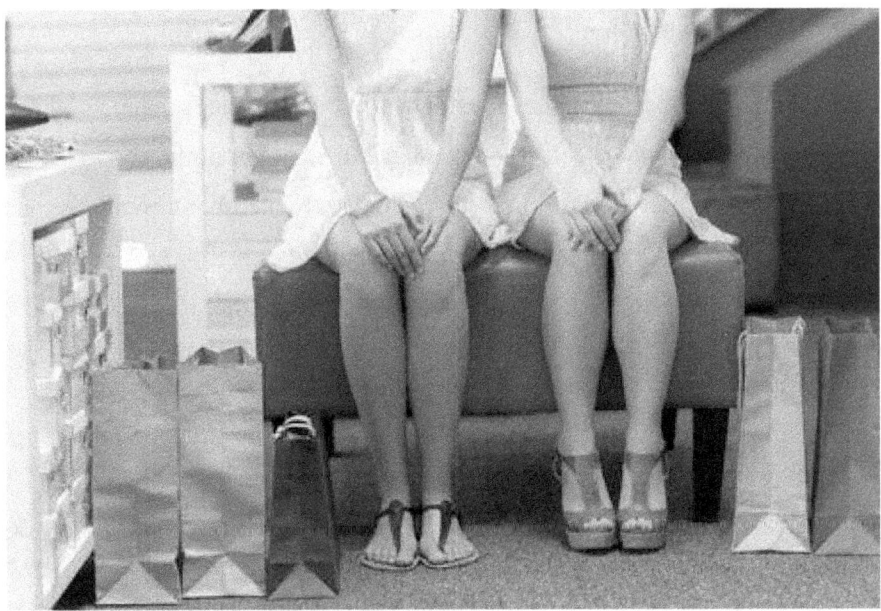

However, in many cases, even if there is nothing lying deep in your subconscious, you are going to buy a pair of shoes not because they are comfortable but because they are irresistible or because they are being sold at a discount! Do not say you have not done that ever. I have done that. You have done that even if you shake your head at the moment in negation. But do not worry, this is a natural, impulsive instinct, especially when a number of us are confronted with the clothes and shoes.

You need to overcome this habit by judging a shoe by its looks alone by making sure that it fits properly.

Do not be in a hurry when testing out a shoe. The shoe salesman may slip your foot into a dainty pair of shoes, and admire your small feet on your ankles as shown off by the design. Take his approval with a pinch of salt, get up and walk around the showroom. See if you can walk properly. See where the shoes pinch.

If they pinch you, when you have just taken a couple of steps, what are they going to do to your poor feet, when you have to walk out of the shop and onto the road? Remove those shoes immediately. Remember to wriggle your toes and make sure that the front portion of your shoes is roomy. You may want to move your foot inside your shoes to make sure that it is spacey

Shoes have to be lightweight. They should have stable and superior design and cushioning. They should also provide your foot with support and stability.

If you are buying leather shoes, choose the perforated varieties. They allow your feet to breathe.

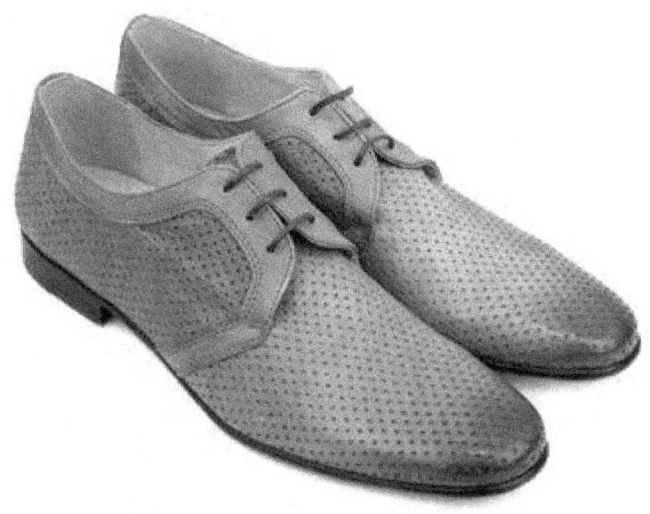

Not being able to find shoes of my size in our particular area, I had to go to one of the well-known shops in the city where the shoes were custom-made. The prices were exorbitant, but we knew that we would get quality goods, because the shop owner took the measure of your foot on a piece of paper.

The shop was recommended to me by my grandmother, because thanks to her bunions, she needed special leather shoes! Well, I was looking at my foot being measured on that piece of paper. The shop owner made sure that her drawing pencil drew the outline of the foot 1 inch away from my foot.

And that is why when the shoes were made up one week afterwards by her experienced workmen, I knew that they would serve me well for a decade or more. This sort of workmanship is getting to be very rare in the world today, but Iris's quality persists to this day, and generations come to her shop as a matter of brand loyalty. Especially as the shop has been in existence for more than 54 years.

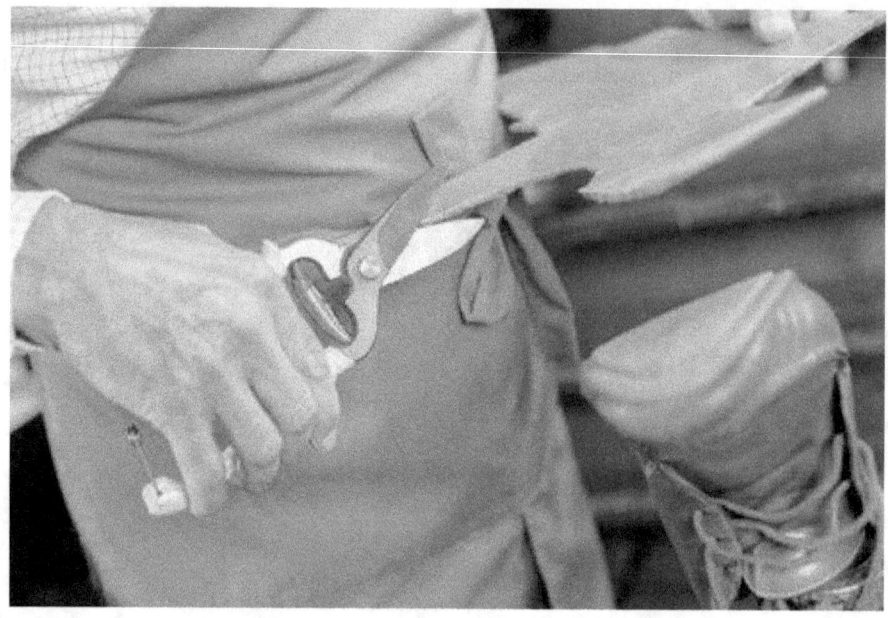

In fact, her shoes have become a brand in our city, and getting shoes from *Sheng's* means that you can afford those shoes and you know quality and style, when you see it. And best of all, you have been handed down a quality shopping experience and heritage from one of your elders who patronized that top-quality shop ages ago!

Remember that the size of your foot is going to attend four – six times even during adulthood. So it is important to get your feet measured every time, whenever you buy a new pair of shoes or get them made up.

The best time to buy shoes is in the evening. That is when your feet have stressed and swollen to their full size.

Natural Footcare

Now that I have told you how you can get rid of foot problems, here are some time tested foot remedies which are going to help you keep your feet soft, silky and healthy.

Oatmeal Scrub

I normally use this scrub for sloughing off dead skin and buffing the dull surfaces of my heels and soles. Mix 1 teaspoon of oatmeal in a cup of water. Dip a fine pumice stone or a sponge in it and scrub away.

Healing Cracked Heels

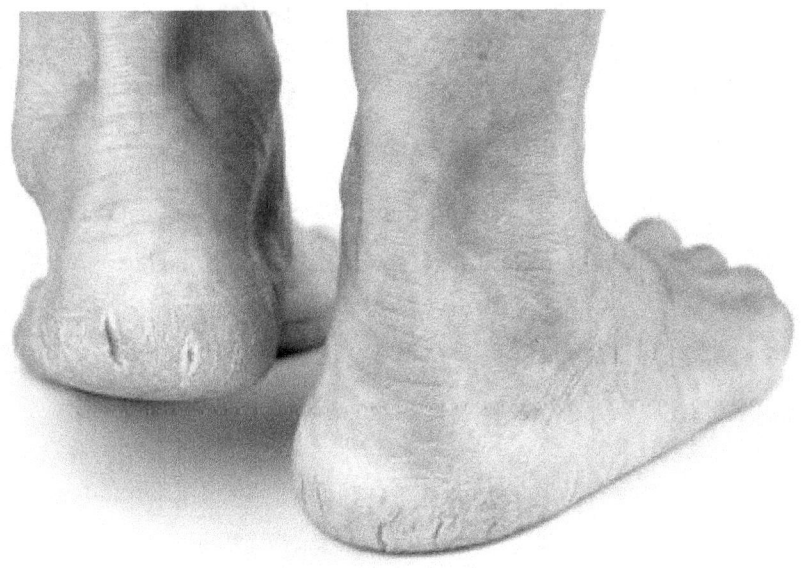

I overheard my grandmother who was rather "With It" describing one of her acquaintances to another of her friends. That particular acquaintance had not managed to overcome her rustic upbringing and background because she had powdered painted and buffed her face and neck beautifully, but she had neglected her cracked heels.

I also remember as a child an aunt telling me, "the sign of good breeding and good blood is seen when you see their feet. They never allow their heels to get chapped."

This meant that that particular person had enough of resources to get servants to massage the heels regularly with olive oil or coconut oil to keep them soft. Also, according to her cracked heels were normally found in people who labored barefoot on land, not worrying about the condition of their feet. They were the ones who had large feet with cracked heels

This was about four decades ago, but that was the social make up of that time.

So if you do not want to be considered a peasant or a rustic, soak your cracked heels in lukewarm water to which you have added a few drops of coconut oil and one teaspoonful of blistering when the water cools down, take out your feet and drive them thoroughly. After that, rub camphor on the heels. This is going to cure the cracks.

When visiting the mountains and the villages there I normally notice the beautiful village women sitting around their fires at night and rubbing their feet with warm coconut oil and mustard oil. After they have sloughed off all the accumulated dust and dirt while massaging their feet, they cover their feet with woolen socks so that the oil does not stain the bed sheets.

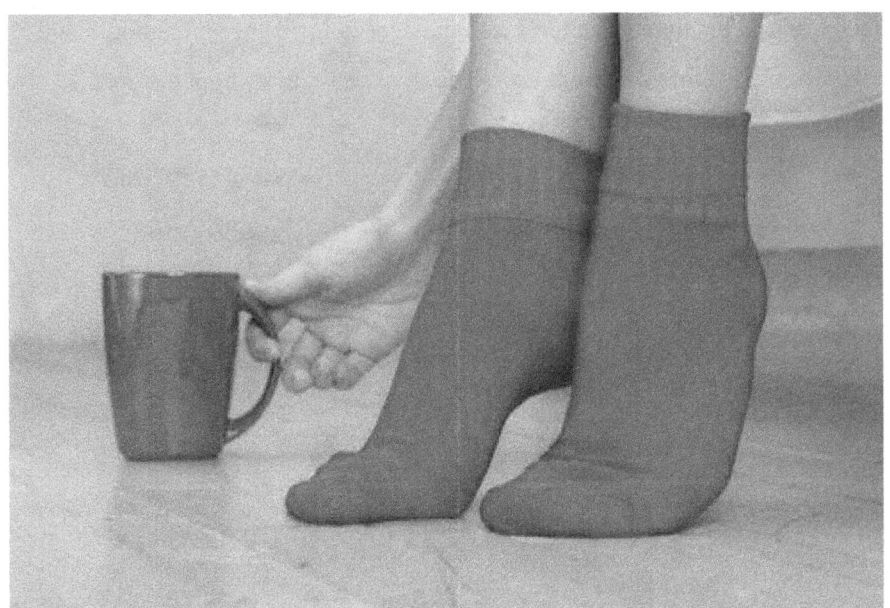

And though they may be called rustic peasants by supercilious snobs, their feet are soft, lovely and dainty, even though they work hard on their land day in day out.

So beautiful feet are not the prerogative of the so-called cultured and educated classes while cracked heels definitely do not belong to the working class alone.

Softening Soles

Here is an excellent way in which you can soften your soles. Just make up a mixture of lemon juice and sugar and rub your soles as well as the other portions of your feet gently with this mixture

You can also get soft feet by soaking them in a mixture of warm water and warm oil. Olive oil, coconut oil and mustard oil is best. Not only are your feet going to be moisturized but also they are going to be soft, smooth and silky, especially after you get rid of the dry skin with a pumice stone.

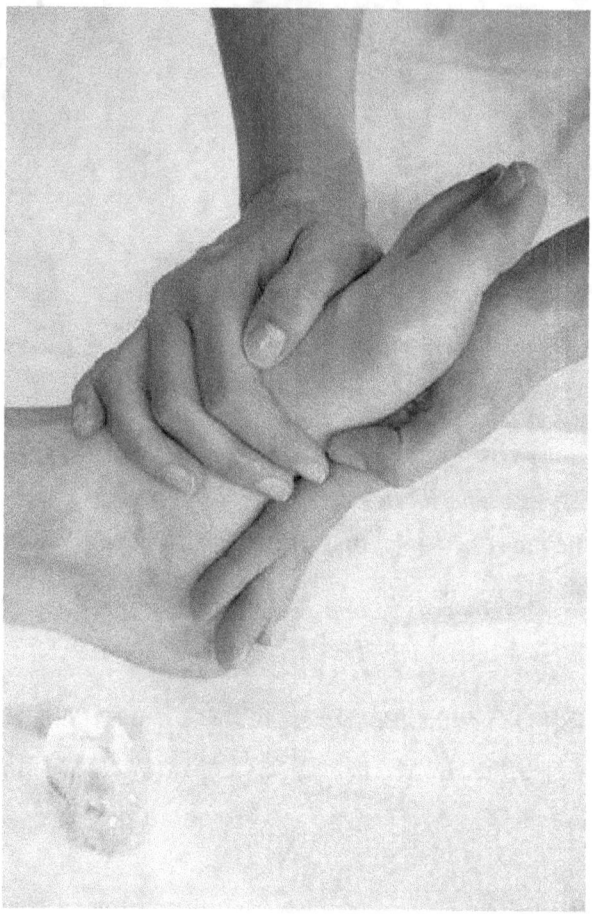

You can also get soft soles by rubbing that area with this scrub of wheat bran and milk.

Conclusion

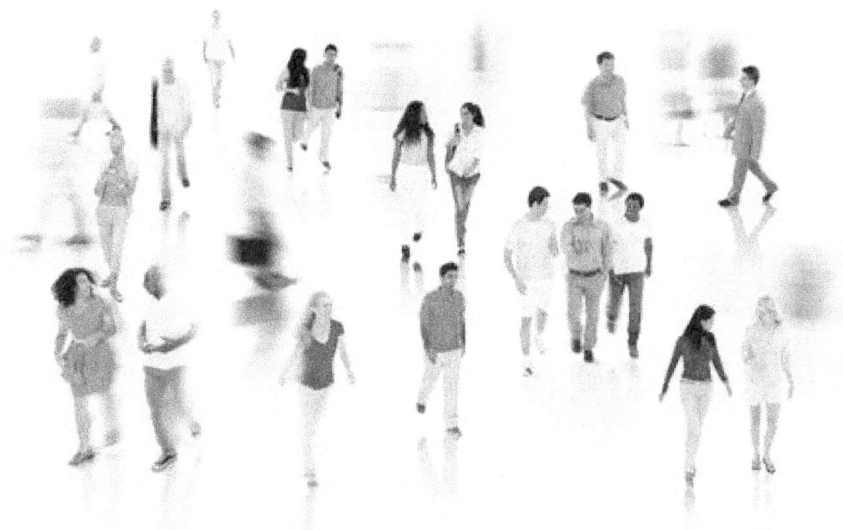

As it has been calculated that feet travel about 70,000 miles in an average lifetime, this book has given you a number of tips and techniques with which you can take care of them. You do not need to suffer from feet problems ever, if you lavish a little bit of care and attention upon them.

If you have to stand for a long time, even if you are wearing sensible shoes, remember to rest your feet, one by one on a small stool. That is so that the blood supply changes direction instead of going downwards in one position for a long while.

Whenever we needed to be given a dressing down or talking to by our drill sergeant on Parade during strenuous physical training sessions, he always made sure that we were at Stand at Ease Position[3] instead of Attention position. That meant that the blood supply to our feet did not cause us to fall down when we were standing too long at one place in one position, and in attention position.

Standing at ease takes off the pressure from your feet. If you have to stand in one position for a long while, do not stand at attention with your feet together. If you have to stand at attention, make sure that the feet are at an angle of 45° from each other with your heels together and your toes pointing outwards.

If your feet are always tired, remember to check your weight. You may be overweight. Put your feet into a tub of lukewarm water containing a cupful of sea salt. This is going to get rid of the aches and pains.

Live Long and Prosper!

---

[3] The moment, he bellowed the command of "stand at ease" after Parade instead of "Dismiss," all of us had an immediate mental reaction of, *oh my God, another half an hour of a Moral Lecture.* Moral lecture stands for a dressing down in army parlay where our iniquities and shortcomings would be described minutely and thoroughly in a highly moral manner and fashion.

Author Bio

Dueep Jyot Singh is a Management and IT Professional who managed to gather Postgraduate qualifications in Management and English and Degrees in Science, French and Education while pursuing different enjoyable career options like being an hospital administrator, IT,SEO and HRD Database Manager/ trainer, movie , radio and TV scriptwriter, theatre artiste and public speaker, lecturer in French, Marketing and Advertising, ex-Editor of Hearts On Fire (now known as Solstice) Books Missouri USA, advice columnist and cartoonist, publisher and Aviation School trainer, ex-moderator on Medico.in, banker, student councilor ,travelogue writer ... among other things!

One fine morning, she decided that she had enough of killing herself by Degrees and went back to her first love -- writing. It's more enjoyable! She already has 48 published academic and 14 fiction- in- different- genre books under her belt.

When she is not designing websites or making Graphic design illustrations for clients , she is browsing through old bookshops hunting for treasures, of which she has an enviable collection – including R.L. Stevenson, O.Henry, Dornford Yates, Maurice Walsh, De Maupassant, Victor Hugo, Sapper, C.N. Williamson, "Bartimeus" and the crown of her collection- Dickens "The Old Curiosity Shop," and "Martin Chuzzlewit" and so on... Just call her "Renaissance Woman") - collecting herbal remedies, acting like Universal Helping Hand/Agony Aunt, or escaping to her dear mountains for a bit of exploring, collecting herbs and plants and trekking.

Check out some of the other JD-Biz Publishing books

Gardening Series on Amazon

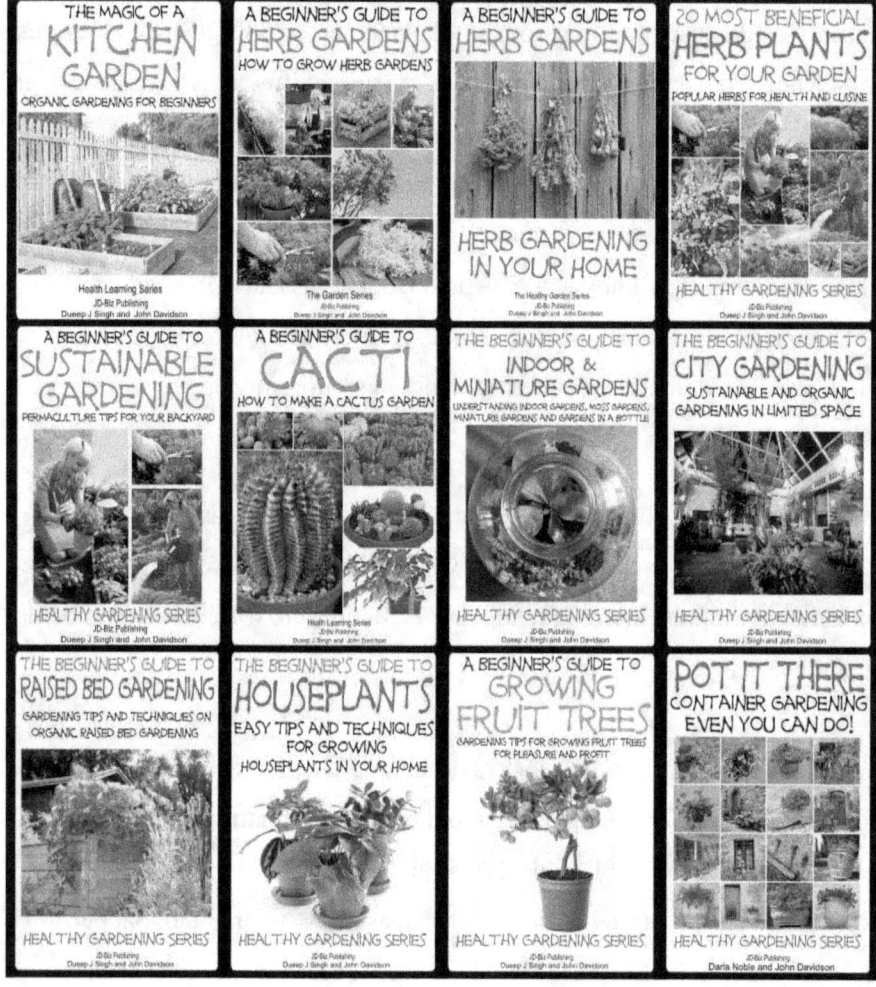

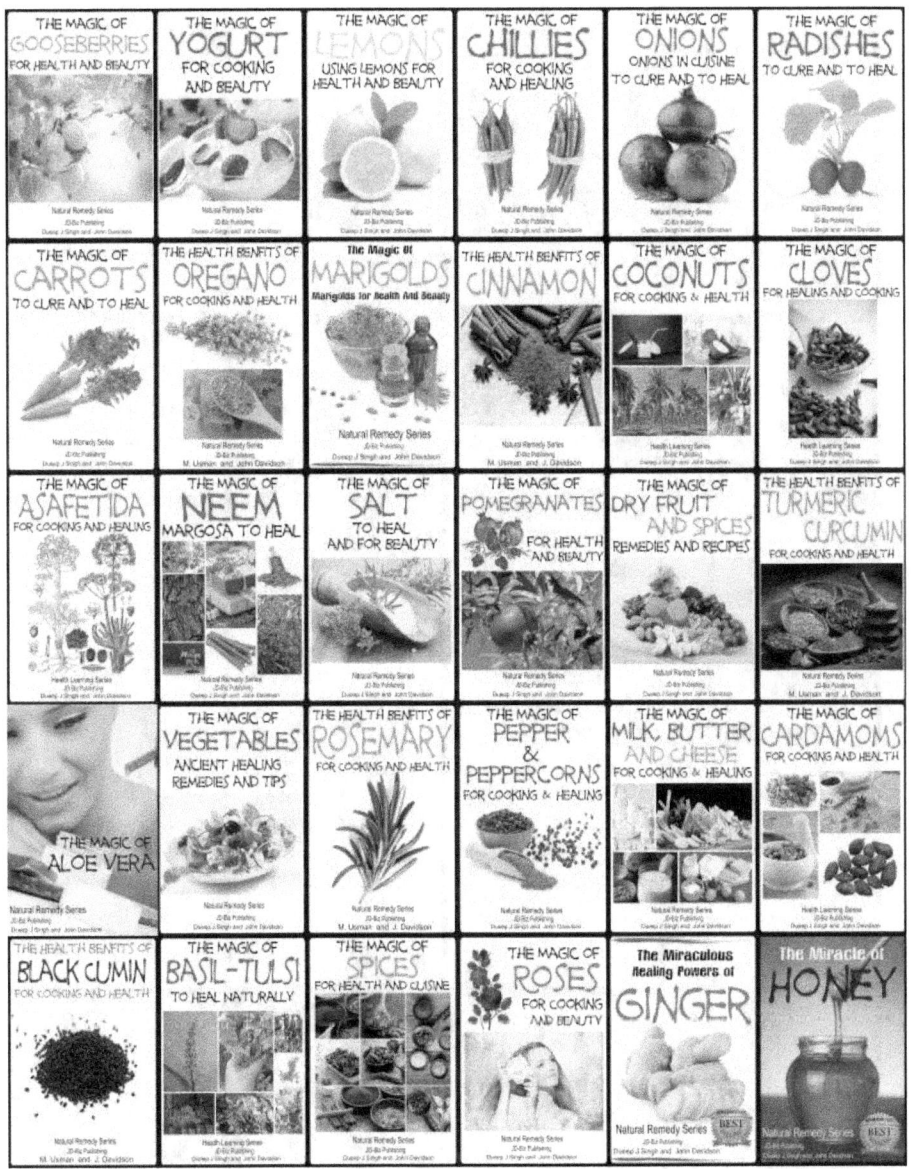

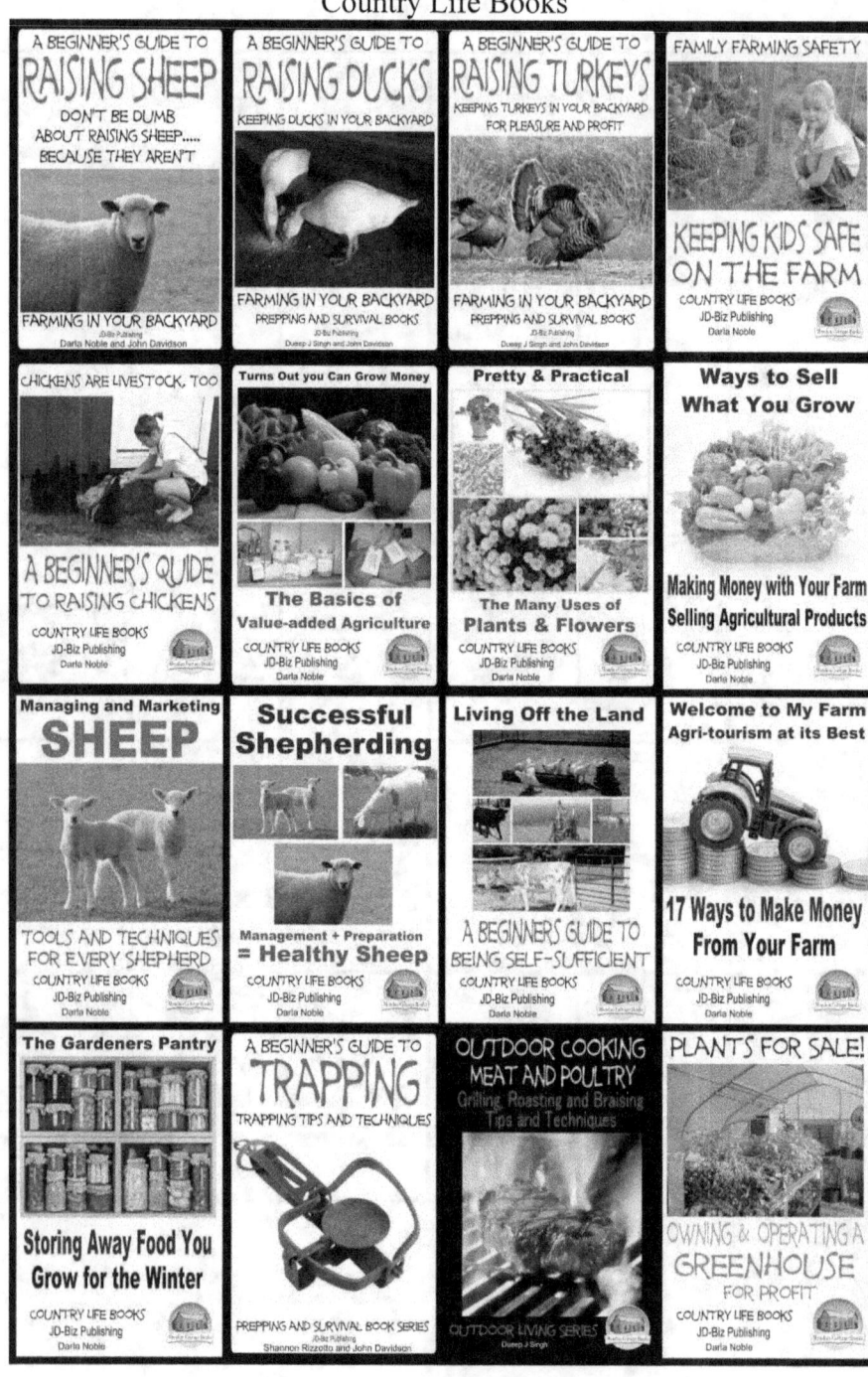

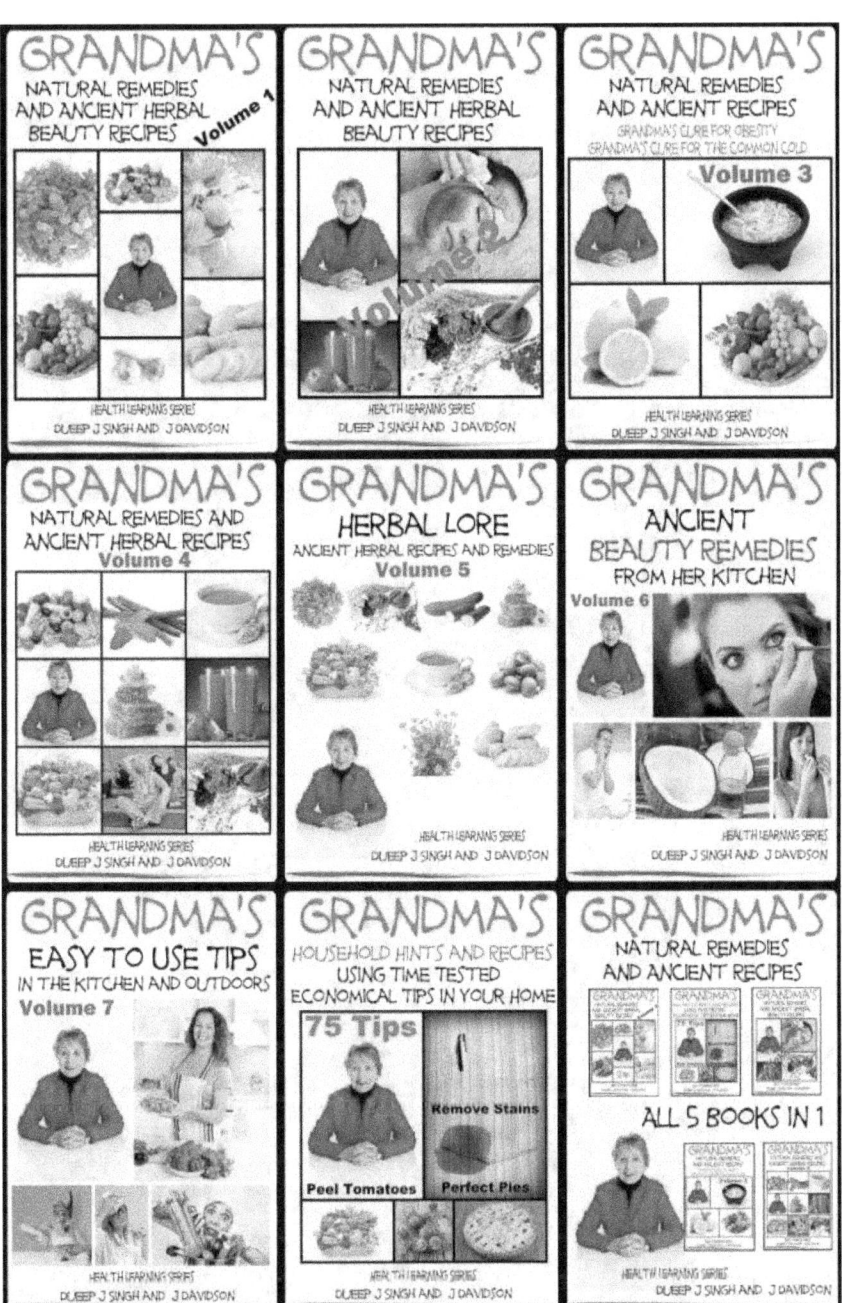

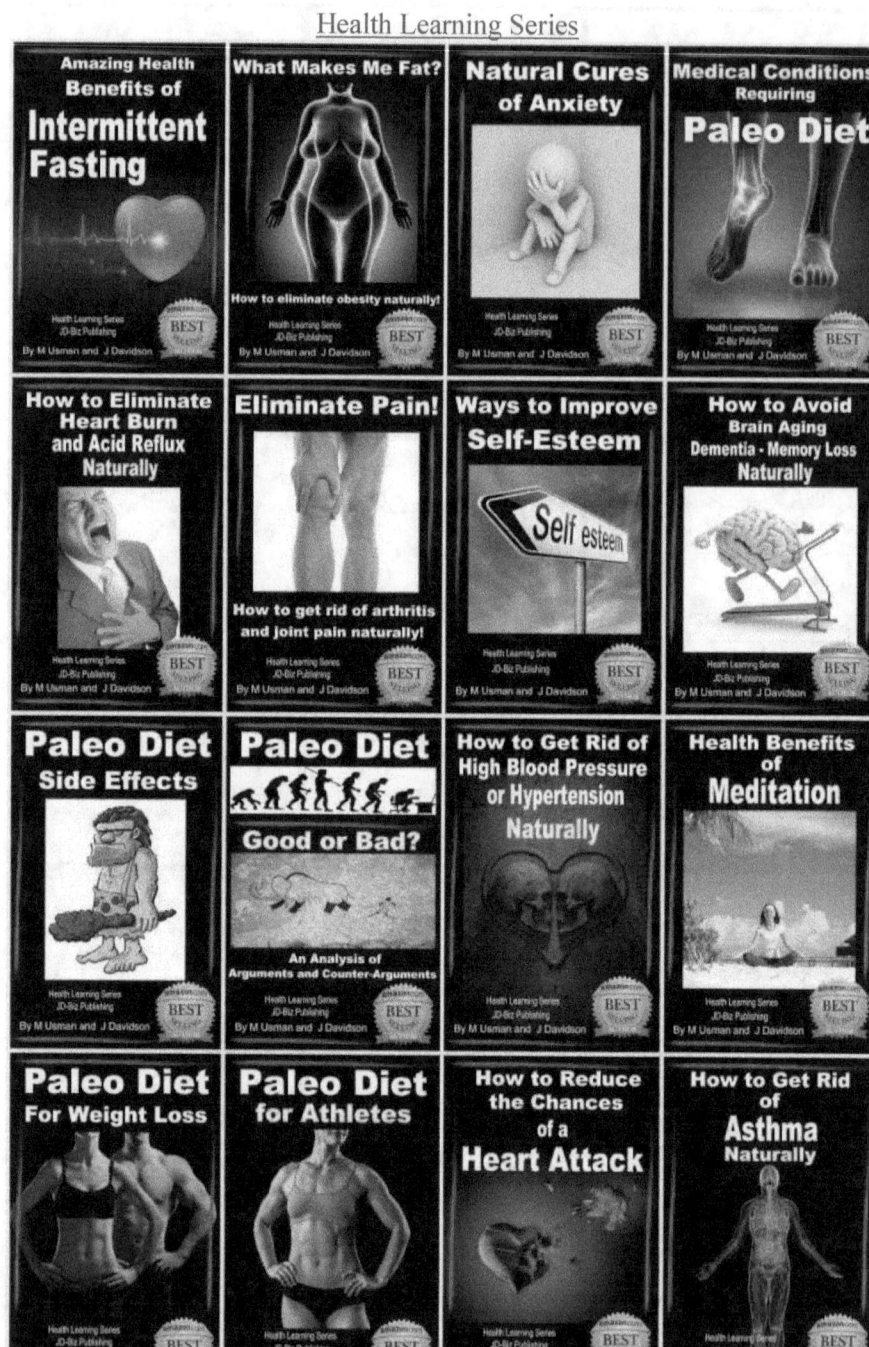

Amazing Animal Book Series

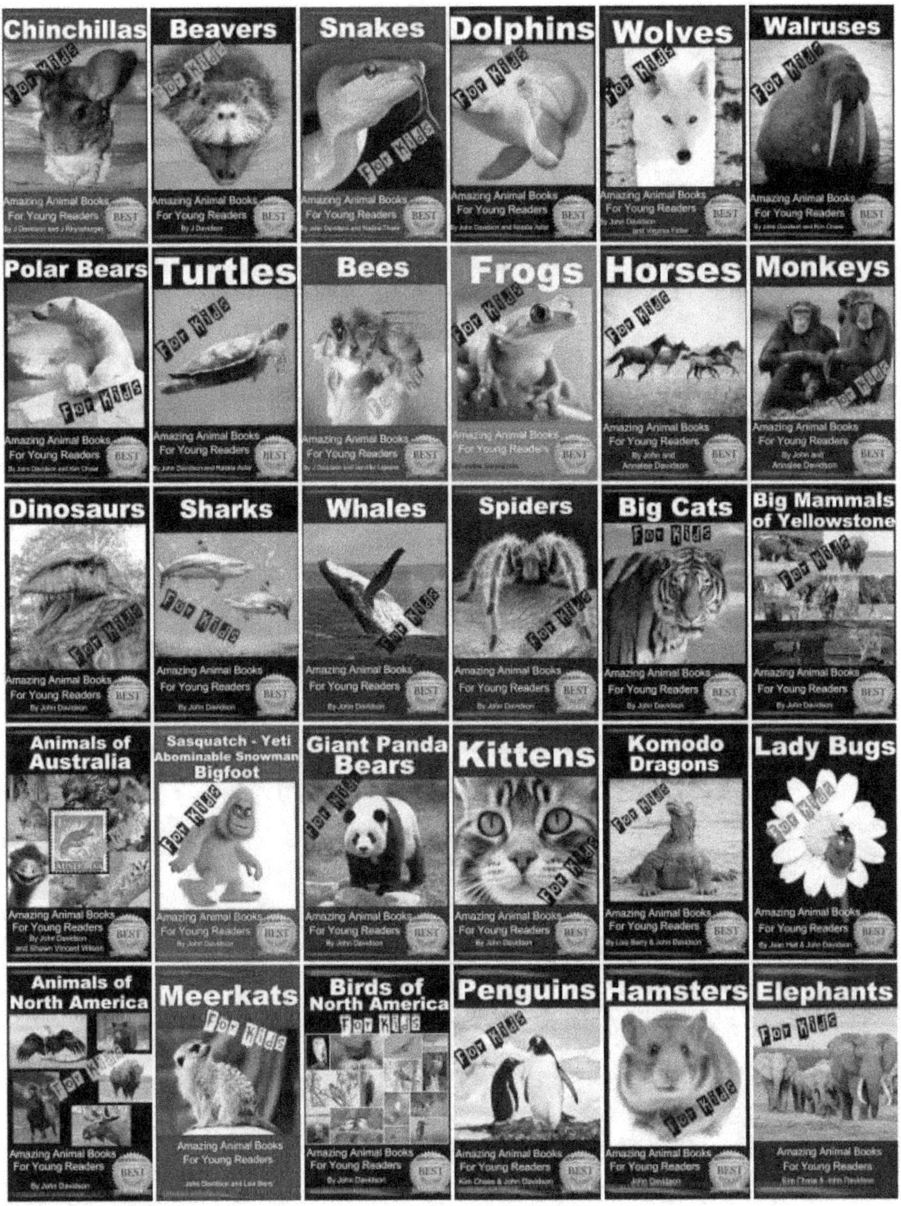

Learn To Draw Series

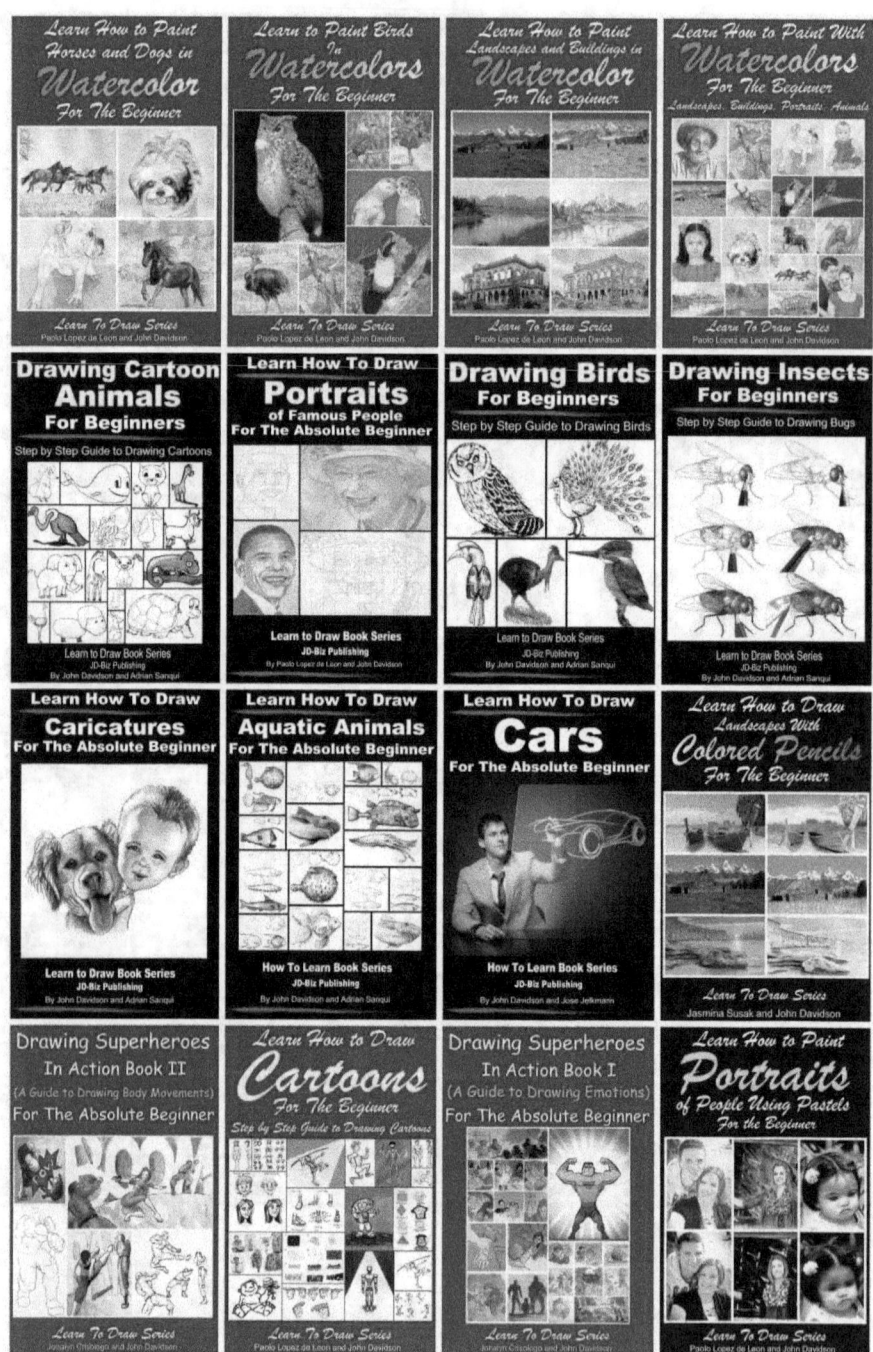

How to Build and Plan Books

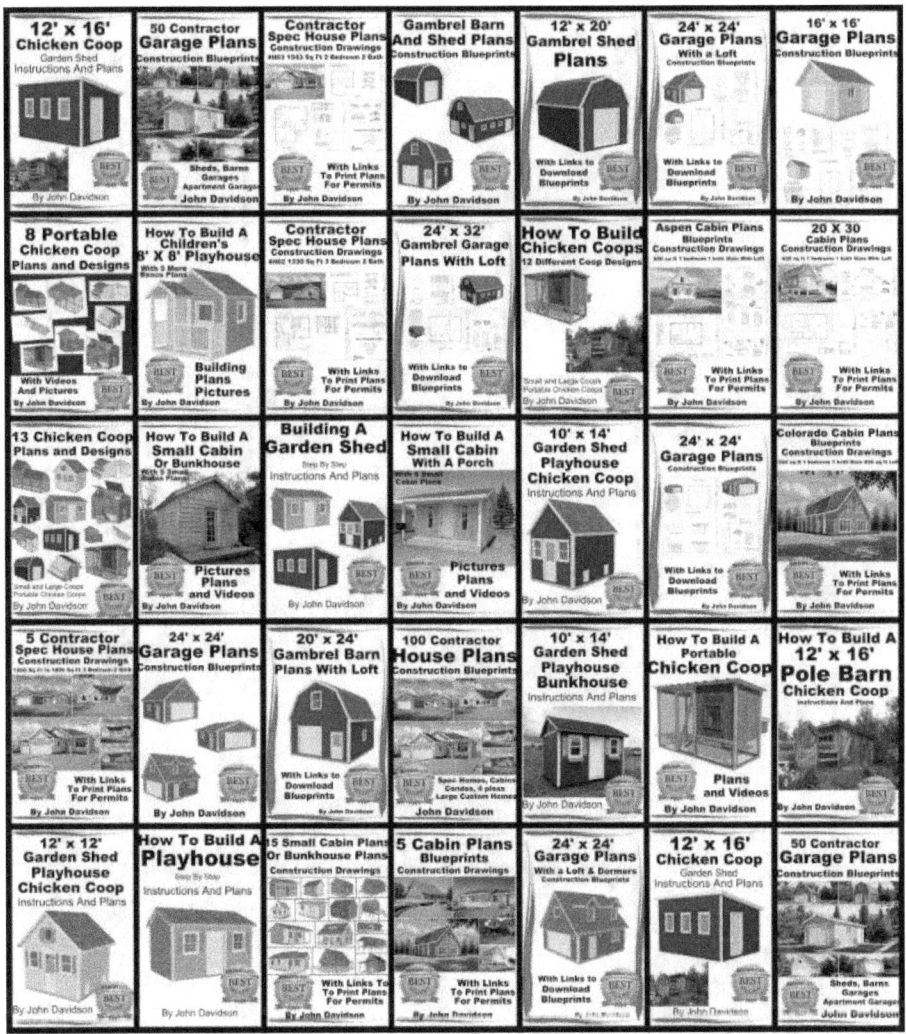

Entrepreneur Book Series

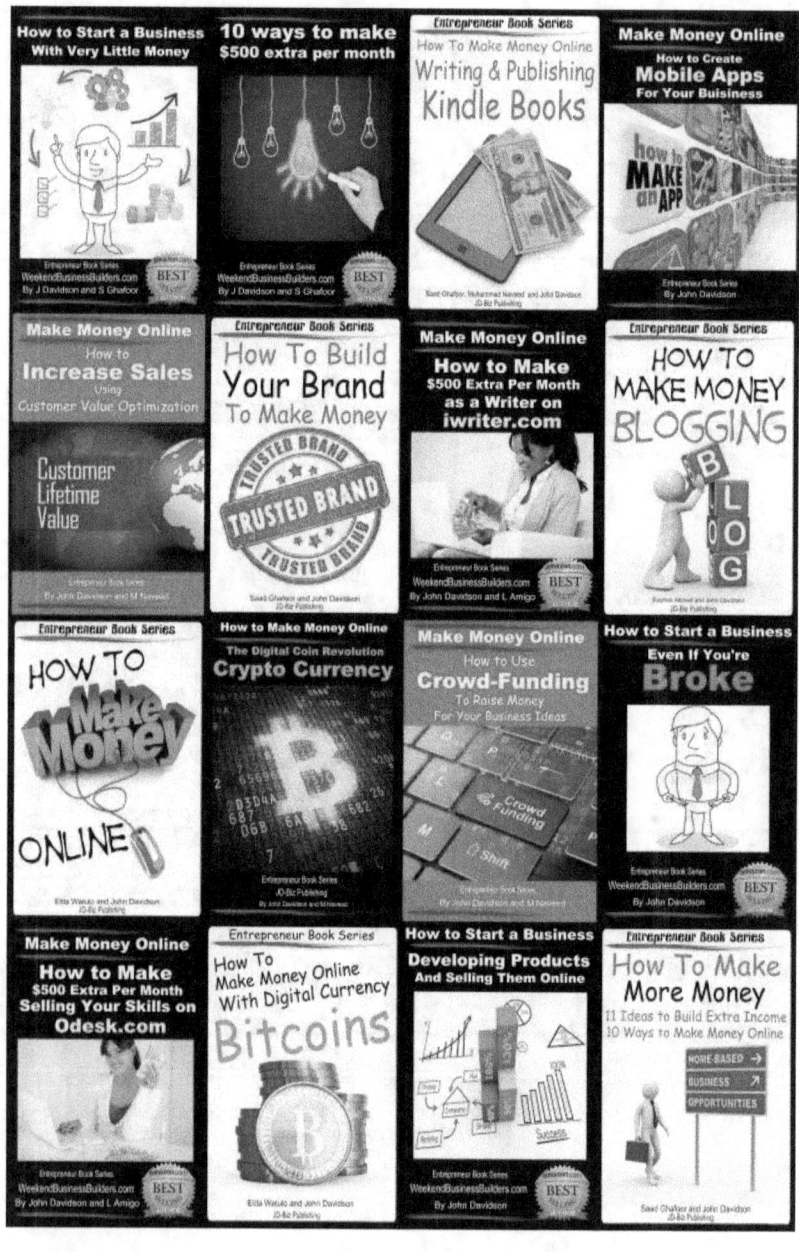

Our books are available at

1. Amazon.com

2. Barnes and Noble

3. Itunes

4. Kobo

5. Smashwords

6. Google Play Books

Publisher

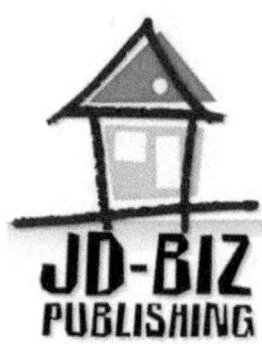

JD-Biz Corp

P O Box 374

Mendon, Utah 84325

http://www.jd-biz.com/

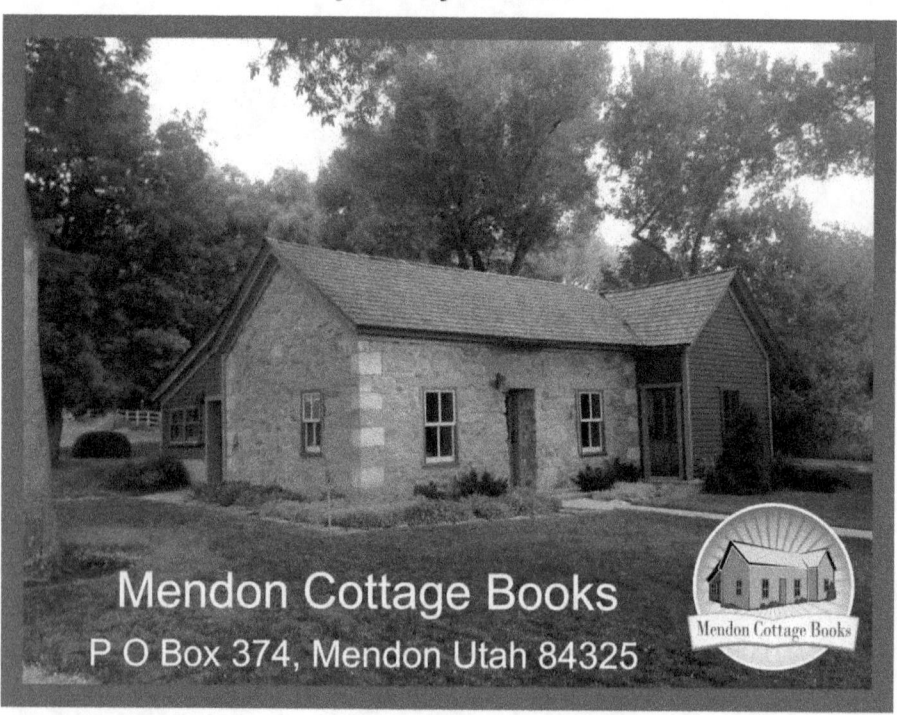